2023 PLANT BASED BUYERS GUIDE

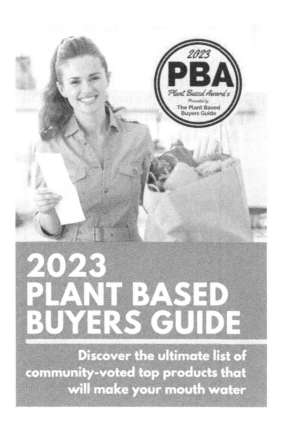

2023
PLANT BASED
BUYERS GUIDE

Discover the ultimate list of
community-voted top products that
will make your mouth water

JOSH SCHIEFFER

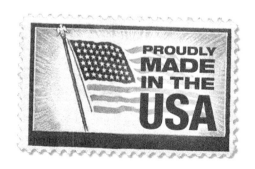

Table of Contents

How to Read

Yogurt

2023 Annual Plant Based Awards

1st Place Winner: Two Good Low-fat Lower Sugar Strawberry Greek Yogurt

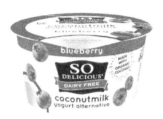

2nd Place Winner: Nancy's Yogurt Apple Cinnamon Probiotic Oat Milk Yogurt

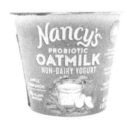

3rd Place Winner: Kite Hill Unsweetened Vanilla Yogurt

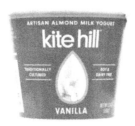

Runner Up:

Forager Project Organic Dairy-Free Strawberry Cashewmilk Yogurt

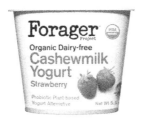

Other Great Products:

Kite Hill Vanilla Protein Yogurt

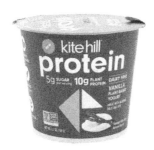

Introduction by Josh Schieffer

This happens to be our 14th year producing consumer-based award programs and we are excited to connect you to the results. If you are not familiar with the guide, I thought it would be best to explain what it is and more importantly what it is not.

This book is not intended for those following a strict vegan diet. <u>Sometimes you will find eggs, honey and other animal products in some of the products listed.</u> The term "Plant-Based Diet" doesn't mean you only eat plants rather your diet is based on consuming mostly plants. Many researchers and dieticians will argue that consuming only plants may lead many to nutrient deficiencies related to vitamin D vitamin B12, calcium, omega-3s, protein and iron if you are not careful. Again, following a vegan diet works from some but we are focusing on products that contain mostly plant-based ingredients. There are currently over 15 different types of veganism and we do not represent any of those types.

Each year, brands and respected plant-based personalities register products into our consumer voting ballot. For a month, we push that ballot to the Plant Based community allowing them to vote for their favorite products on the ballot. We publish the buyers guide with the award results organized by category. Nothing fancy, just consumers helping consumers, the way it should be.

This book is much more than a list of great plant based products to buy, we also list some of the best plant based personalities. Being on a plant based diet can be isolating in so many ways and difficult at first.

This book does not contain every single plant based product available in every market. The food industry has changed dramatically since we started in 2008. Virtually no regional grocery chains had private label plant based products and now it is the norm with west coast chains like Safeway and east coast chains like Publix. We tend to focus on brands with national distribution and national grocery chains. We do this so you have access to these products regardless of where you live. Oftentimes ordering online can save you money, time and widen your options dramatically.

You will not find every brand or product listed in this book on your local grocery shelves. It's a strange fact to some but often brands must pay to sit on the shelves of most grocery stores. This is especially true for products that don't get purchased as often, like plant based products. If you have a favorite product that your store doesn't carry, you can request that they stock it for a trial period. If it sells, more than likely they will keep it without the brand paying for the space. However, if a competing brand buys out the shelf space your product will more than likely disappear. This is the cold hard truth about the industry. Those who eat plant based food to maintain a healthy lifestyle ultimately pay the price. Oftentimes plant based food is medicine for a diagnosis or health situation we didn't want or ask for. Please use this guide to help make your plant based lifestyle the best it can be.

Why do I tell you all of this? Those of us with restricted diets have limited options especially in rural parts of the country. I do not want your diet and the products you eat being dictated by what brands pay to sit on your local shelves. The product placement in your local store is not based on how great the product is and how well it tastes. If you want to have the best plant based products in your pantry, more than likely you will need to travel to multiple stores and order online.

At the end of the day, I want you to know that there are great plant based products for you. If you are new to the plant based diet or just struggling to maintain the diet because of product availability or poor product quality, we published this book for you. Please read "Our Story" so you have a better understanding of why we have hundreds of product pictures and not just a list of a million random plant based products.

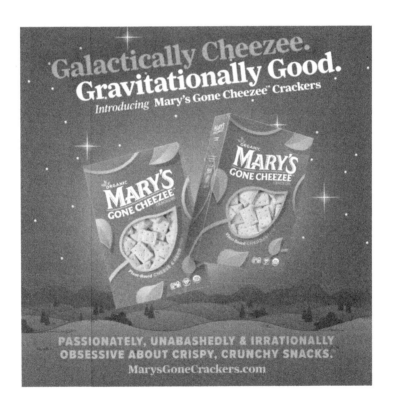

MAKES DINNER
CHEF'S KISS

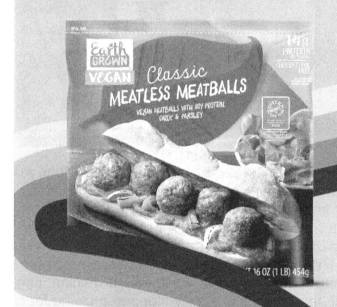

It's an thing.

Our Story

The story behind The Guided Buyer that very few people know

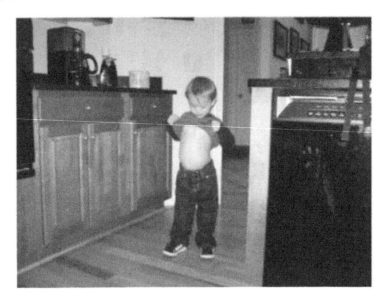

I remember it like it was yesterday when my four-year-old son Jacob, now seventeen, was playing in the kiddie pool with other kids that I assumed were his age based on their height. After asking all the surrounding kids what ages they were, I realized Jacob was significantly smaller than kids his own age. This prompted my wife and I to seek a professional opinion. After consulting with our family physician, she confirmed that Jacob had essentially stopped growing for an entire year without us realizing it. He was referred to Jeff Gordon's Children's Hospital in Charlotte North Carolina to discuss possible growth hormone therapy. The doctors there reviewed Jacob's case and requested a few blood tests based on some suspicions they had.

Our cell phone service at our house was terrible so when the doctor finally called with the blood results, my wife and I ran to the front of the driveway to hear the doctor clearly. With a sporadic signal, we heard "Jacob has celiac disease." We looked at each other as tears ran down my wife's face. We huddled closer to the phone and asked, "what is celiac disease?". After getting a brief description mixed with crappy cell service and happy neighbors waving as they drove by, my wife and I embraced and wept. We were told to maintain his normal diet until we could have an endoscopy and biopsy for further confirmation. Once confirmed our next visit was to a registered dietitian for guidance.

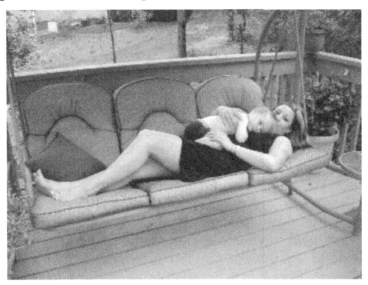

Jayme, my wife, made the appointment and called me with a weird request. "Will you meet me at the dietitian's house for a consultation?". I was confused when she said to go to her house. Jayme then explained that the dietician's daughter had celiac disease too and the best way to show the new lifestyle to patients would be to dive right in. I'll admit, it was a bit uncomfortable at first to be in a strangers' house looking at their personal items but looking back now, I wouldn't change it for the world. That encounter is ultimately the motivation behind the consumer awards and the associated buyers guides. We left her house with complete understanding of best practices and what products they personally liked and disliked. That visit was life changing and left us feeling confident as we made our way to the local health food store.

That first trip shopping took forever. Each label was read, and cross checked with our list of known gluten containing suspects. It was also shocking to see the bill when it was time to pay. We had replaced our entire pantry and fridge with all products that had the "gluten-free" label. We both worked full-time and had decent paying jobs and it still set us back financially.

We looked for support groups locally and came across a "100% Gluten-Free Picnic" in Raleigh, which was two hours away from where we lived. This was our first time meeting other people with celiac disease and we were fortunate to have met some informative people that were willing to help with the hundreds of questions we had. We were introduced to a family whose son had been recently diagnosed with celiac disease as well. His condition was much worse than Jacobs and he was almost hospitalized before finally being diagnosed. They confided in us as we shared similar stories. There were two key differences that would light a motivational fire I could not extinguish. The first was the fact that they didn't have the same experience with a registered dietitian. Instead, they were handed a two-page Xerox copy of "safe foods". Second, they didn't have the financial security to experiment with gluten-free counterparts. Their first two months exposed to the gluten free lifestyle left them extremely depressed and financially broke.

On our way home from that picnic, Jayme and I felt compelled to help make a difference in some way. We were determined to help that family and others being diagnosed with this disease. Up until that day, we hadn't found a resource that gave unbiased opinions on gluten free products and services. Fast forward a few years and I too was diagnosed with celiac disease. That year, The Gluten-Free Awards were born.

Originally our vision was to create a one-page website with a handful of categories organized by peoples' favorites. Each year we grew; more products, more categories, and eventually a buyers guide by request. For years we had been asked to produce similar programs and buyer guides for other diets. In 2020 we expanded yet again with adding three new diets to our consumer awards programs. We now host:

The Gluten Free Awards & Buyers Guide

The Plant Based Awards & Buyers Guide

The Low-Carb Awards & Buyers Guide

The Dairy Free Awards & Buyers Guide

We want to thank those special people and organizations that brought us to where we are today:

Pat Fogarty MS, RD, LDN for allowing us to enter your home.

Jeff Gordon's Children's Hospital

Raleigh Celiac Support Groups

Dean Meisel, MD, FAAP for the excellent medical care he provides for our family.

I hope you have learned something new from the story behind The Guided Buyer. Today, Jacob and I continue to live a healthy lifestyle.

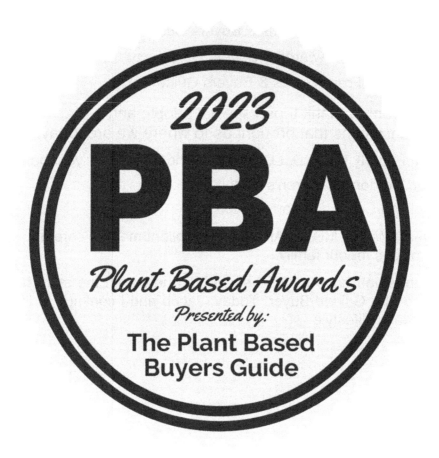

Bread & Bakery

Bagels

2023 Annual Plant Based Awards

1st Place Winner: Dave's Killer Bread Plain Awesome Bagels

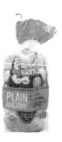

2nd Place Winner: 365 by Whole Foods Market Plain Bagels

3rd Place Winner: Canyon Bakehouse Everything Bagels

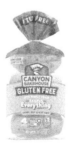

Runner Up:

ODoughs Bagel Thins

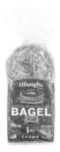

Other Great Bagels:

Bfree Gluten Free Plain Bagels

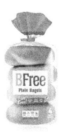

Little Northern Bakehouse Blueberry Bagels

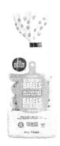

Bread

2023 Annual Plant Based Awards

1st Place Winner: Food For Life Ezekiel 4:9 Flourless Sprouted Grain Bread

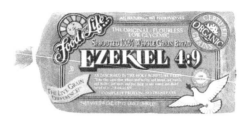

2nd Place Winner: Eatsane Nuts and Seeds Bread Loaf

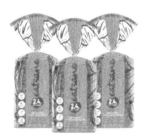

3rd Place Winner: Silver Hills Squirrelly Bread Made with Organic Sprouted Grains

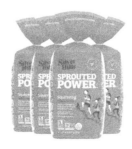

Runner Up:

Outside The Breadbox Vegan Oat Bread

Other Great Breads:

Angel's Bakery Classic White Pita Pillows

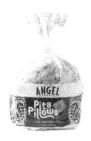

Breadcrumbs

2023 Annual Plant Based Awards

1st Place Winner: Cauli Crunch Original Plant Based Cauli-flower Crumbs

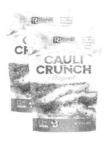

.2nd Place Winner: Carrington Farms Gluten Free Bread Crumbs - Plain

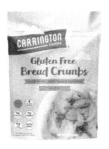

3rd Place Winner: Pereg Panko Japanese Style Toasted Bread Crumbs - Thai Sweet Chilli Flavor

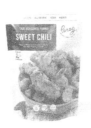

Runner Up:

Yez! Foods Artisan Keto Bread Crumbs

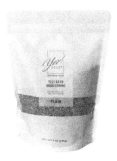

Other Great Products:

Outside the Breadbox Vegan Breadcrumbs

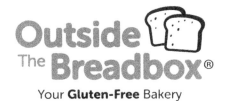

Buns

2023 Annual Plant Based Awards

1st Place Winner: Schar Hamburger Buns

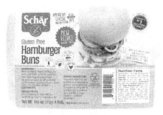

2nd Place Winner: 365 by Whole Food Market Hamburger Buns

3rd Place Winner: Angelic Bakehouse Slider Buns

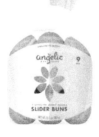

Runner Up:

Happy Campers Wild Gluten Free Hamburger Buns

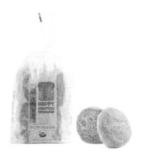

Other Great Buns:

Outside The Breadbox Buns

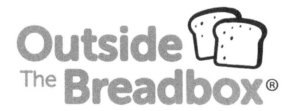

Cookies

2023 Annual Plant Based Awards

1st Place Winner: Siete Family Foods Mexican Shortbread Cookie

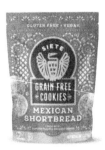

2nd Place Winner: PARTAKE FOODS Crunchy Chocolate Chip Cookies

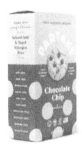

3rd Place Winner: ALDI-exclusive Simply Nature Vanilla Coconut Cashew Crisps

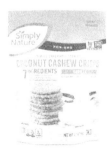

Runner Up:

ALDI-exclusive Simply Nature Salted Caramel Coconut Cashew Crisps

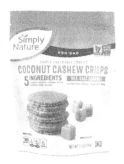

Other Great Products:

ALDI-exclusive Simply Nature Chocolate Coconut Cashew Crisps

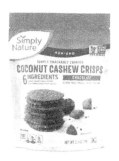

Lucy's Chocolate Chip

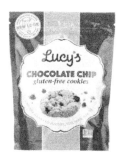

Pizza Crust

2022 Annual Plant Based Awards

1st Place Winner: Uncrust by Unbun

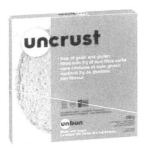

2nd Place Winner: Cappello's, Naked Pizza Crust

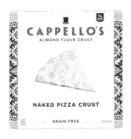

3rd Place Winner: BFree Stone Baked Pizza Crust

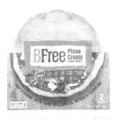

Runner Up:

Banza Plain Chickpea Pizza Crust

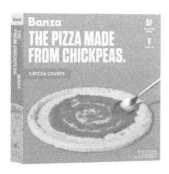

Other Great Products:

Trader Joe's Cauliflower Crust

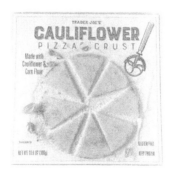

Rolls

2022 Annual Plant Based Awards

1st Place Winner: ThinSlim Foods Rustic Tuscan Olive and Garlic Rolls

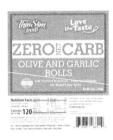

2nd Place Winner: Keto Factory Cinnamon Rolls Mix

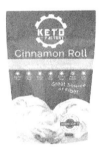

3rd Place Winner: Ener-G Gluten Free Keto Rolls

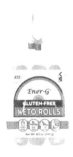

DELICIOUSLY SWEET, DECADENT, & GLUTEN-FREE

It's so good that you won't want to share it!

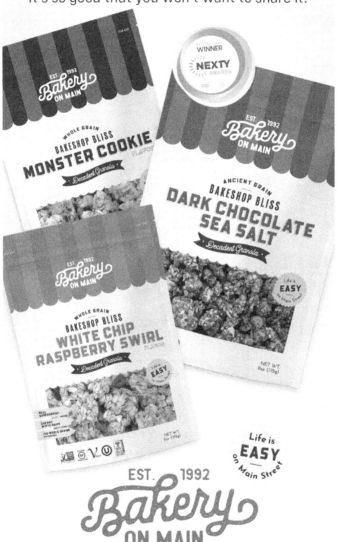

Tortilla

2023 Annual Plant Based Awards

1st Place Winner: Siete Family Foods Cassava Chia Tortilla

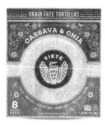

2nd Place Winner: Caulipower Tortilla Cauliflower

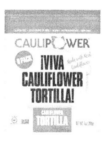

3rd Place Winner: MARIA & RICARDOS Quinoa Flour Tortillas

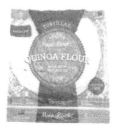

Runner Up:

Mi Rancho Organic Corn Tortillas

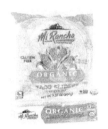

Other Great Products:

Mission Cauliflower Tortillas

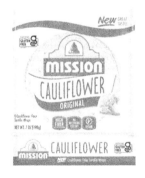

Wrap

2023 Annual Plant Based Awards

1st Place Winner: NASOYA FOODS Wonton Wraps

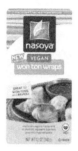

2nd Place Winner: Angelic Bakehouse Turmeric Sweet Potato Garden Wraps

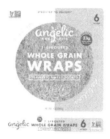

3rd Place Winner: TaDah! Falafel Wrap Lemony Garlic Hummus

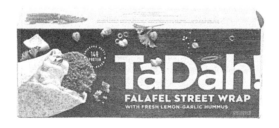

Runner Up:

Raw Wraps Kale Wraps

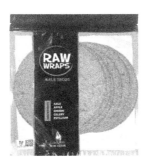

Other Great Products:

Mission Garden Spinach Wraps

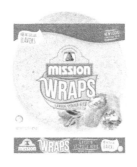

Breakfast

Breakfast On-The-Go

2023 Annual Plant Based Awards

1st Place Winner: Catalina Crunch Chocolate Peanut Butter Keto Cereal

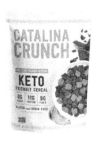

2nd Place Winner: YES Bar – Salted Maple Pecan – Decadent Snack Bar

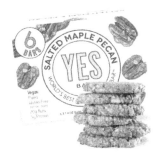

3rd Place Winner: Alpha Foods Breakfast Burrito

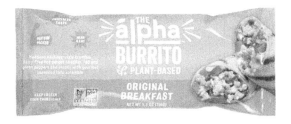

Runner Up:

Alpha Foods Breakfast Sandwich

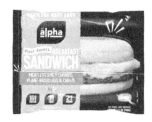

Other Great Products:

KIND Breakfast Bars

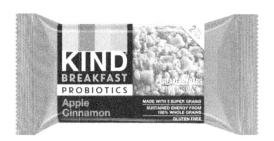

Cold Cereals

2023 Annual Plant Based Awards

1st Place Winner: Nature's Path Organic Panda Puffs Cereal

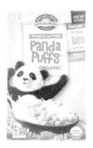

2nd Place Winner: Seven Sundays Berry Grain Free Cereal

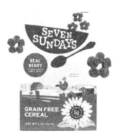

3rd Place Winner: CATALINA SNACKS INC Cinnamon Toast Cereal

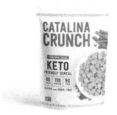

Runner Up:

Three Wishes Cereal Cinnamon Grain Free Cereal

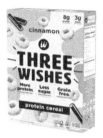

Other Great Products:

Love Grown Power O's Cinnamon Cereal

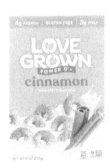

Donuts

2023 Annual Plant Based Awards

1st Place Winner: Krispy Kreme Vegan Donuts

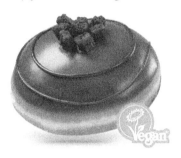

2nd Place Winner: The Vegan Knife Gluten Free & Vegan Cinnamon Sugar Donut Baking Mix

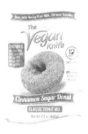

3rd Place Winner: Whole Foods Market Plain Donut Katz

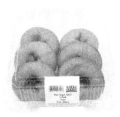

Runner Up:

Gluten Free Powdered Donuts

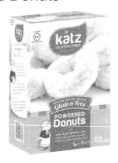

Other Great Products:

Katz Gluten Free Sea Salt Caramel Donuts

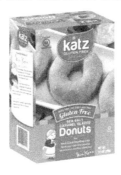

Frozen Pancake & Waffle Brands

2023 Annual Plant Based Awards

1st Place Winner: Nature's Path Organic Dark Chocolate Chip Waffles

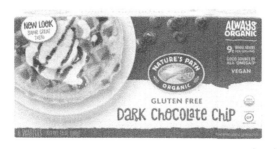

2nd Place Winner: Birch Benders Paleo Toaster Waffles

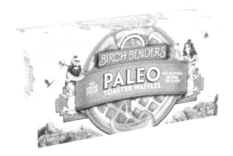

3rd Place Winner: 365 by Whole Foods Market Frozen Organic Pancakes - Multigrain

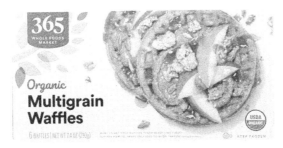

Runner Up:

LIBERATED Paleo Waffles

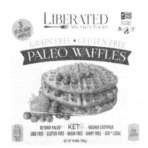

Other Great Products:

Vans Blueberry Power Grains Waffles

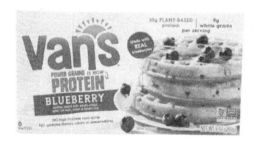

Pancake and Waffle Mixes

2023 Annual Plant Based Awards

1st Place Winner: Better Batter Pancake and Biscuit Mix

2nd Place Winner: Birch Benders Plant Protein Pancake & Waffle Mix

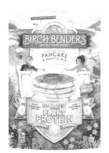

3rd Place Winner: gfJules Gluten Free Pancake & Waffle Mix

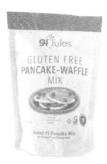

Runner Up:

Pamela's Pancake & Baking Mix

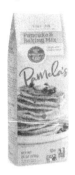

Other Great Products:

Thrive Switch Pancake and Waffle Mix

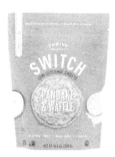

Yogurt

2023 Annual Plant Based Awards

1st Place Winner: So Delicious Yogurt Blueberry

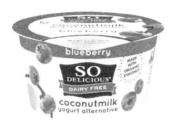

2nd Place Winner: Kite Hill Unsweetened Vanilla Yogurt

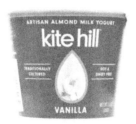

3rd Place Winner: Forager Project Organic Dairy-Free Strawberry Cashewmilk Yogurt

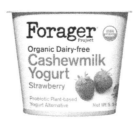

Runner Up:

Harmless Harvest Strawberry Coconut Yogurt

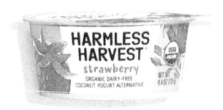

Other Great Products:

Nancy's Yogurt Apple Cinnamon Probiotic Oat Milk Yogurt

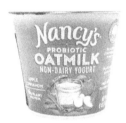

Kite Hill Vanilla Protein Yogurt

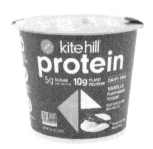

Cookies, Snacks & Candy

Candy

2023 Annual Plant Based Awards

1st Place Winner: UNREAL Dark Chocolate Peanut Butter Cups

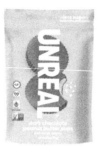

2nd Place Winner: YumEarth Organic Giggles Chewy Candy

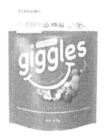

3rd Place Winner: Blissfully Better Dark Chocolate Bon Bons

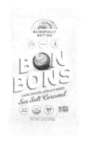

Runner Up:

Hu Simple Dark Chocolate Bars

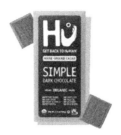

Other Great Products:

Lovely Co. Chewy Candies

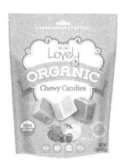

Smart Sweets Sour Blast Buddies

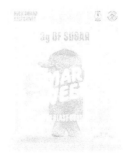

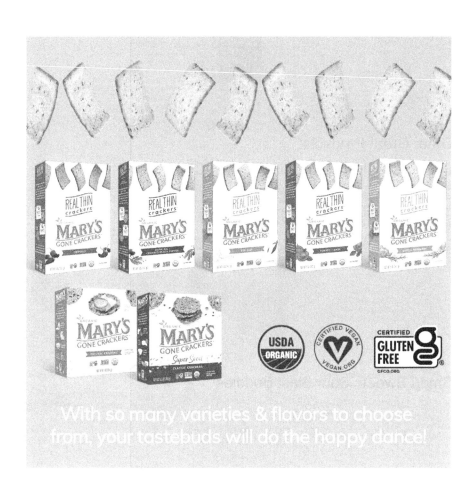

With so many varieties & flavors to choose from, your tastebuds will do the happy dance!

Chips

2023 Annual Plant Based Awards

1st Place Winner: Terra Chips Blue Potato Chips

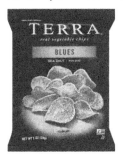

2nd Place Winner: Siete Family Foods Nacho Tortilla Chips

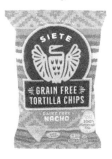

3rd Place Winner: ALDI-exclusive Simply Nature Black Bean Chips

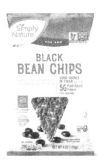

Runner Up:

Brad's Plant Based Sweet Potato Chips

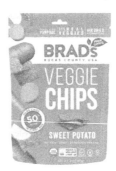

Other Great Products:

Enjoy Life Lentil Chips – Garlic and Parmesan

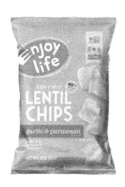

Crackers

2023 Annual Plant Based Awards

1st Place Winner: Mary's Gone Crackers Original

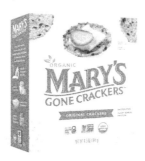

2nd Place Winner: Mary's Gone Crackers REAL Thin Garlic + Rosemary

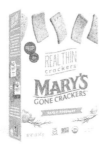

3rd Place Winner: ALDI-exclusive Simply Nature Sea Salt Cauliflower Crackers

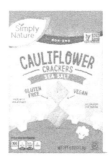

Runner Up:

ALDI-exclusive Simply Nature Cheddar Cauliflower Crackers

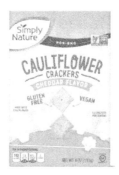

Other Great Products:

Mary's Gone Crackers Super Seed Classic

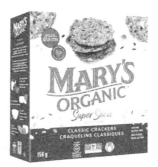

Mary's Gone Crackers REAL Thin Olive Oil + Cracked Black Pepper

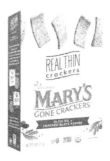

Mary's Gone Crackers REAL Thin Chipotle

Mary's Gone Crackers REAL Thin Tomato + Basil

Granola

2023 Annual Plant Based Awards

1st Place Winner: Bakery On Main Ancient Grain Cranberry Almond Maple Granola

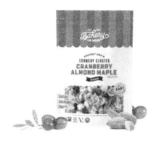

2nd Place Winner: Purely Elizabeth Original Ancient Grain Granola

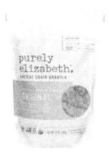

3rd Place Winner: Pure Bliss Organics Naughty But Nice Granola

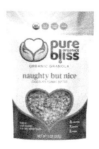

Runner Up:

Michele's Granola Original Granola

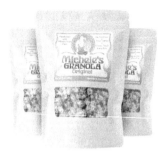

Other Great Products:

One Degree Organic Foods Quinoa Cacao Granola

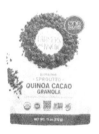

Jerky

2023 Annual Plant Based Awards

1st Place Winner: Louisville Vegan Jerky Co. Carolina Bbq Jerky

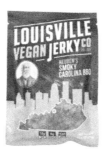

2nd Place Winner: Noble Jerky – Teriyaki

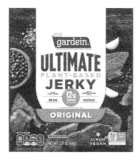

3rd Place Winner: Gardein Ultimate Plant-Based Jerky - Original

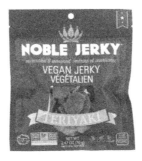

Runner Up:

Electric Jerky - Texas BBQ

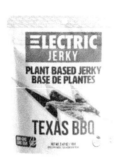

Other Great Products:

Pan's Mushroom Jerky – Original

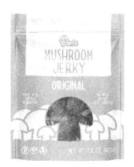

KRAVE Korean BBQ Plant-Based Jerky

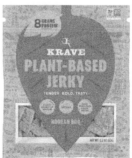

Munchies

2023 Annual Plant Based Awards

1st Place Winner: Mary's Gone Crackers REAL Thin Sea Salt

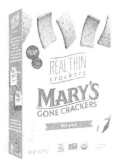

2nd Place Winner: Quinn Snacks Classic Sea Salt Pretzels

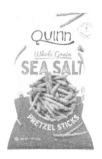

3rd Place Winner: Rhythm Superfoods Organic Buffalo Ranch Cauliflower Bites

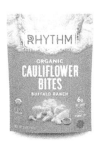

Runner Up:

Skinny Pop White Cheddar

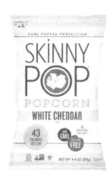

Other Great Products:

Hippeas Organic Chickpea Puffs – White Cheddar

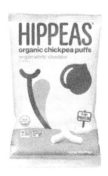

Pretzels

2023 Annual Plant Based Awards

1st Place Winner: Snyder's of Hanover Gluten Free Pretzel Sticks

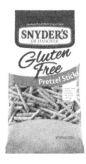

2nd Place Winner: Quinn Snacks Classic Sea Salt Pretzels

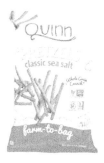

3rd Place Winner: From The Ground Up CAULIFLOWER PRETZEL TWISTS

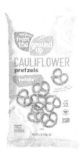

Runner Up:

Unique Pretzel Unique Original Pretzel Splits

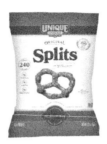

Other Great Products:

Fit Joy Grain Free Pretzel Sticks

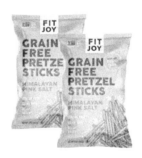

Snack Bars

2023 Annual Plant Based Awards

1st Place Winner: BeBOLD Bars Chocolate Chip Almond Butter

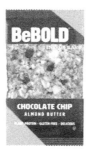

2nd Place Winner: Nature's Bakery Raspberry Fig Bars

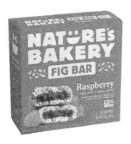

3rd Place Winner: Bobo's Oat Bars Oat Bars Coconut

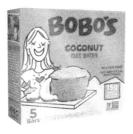

Runner Up:

Good To Go Double Chocolate Soft Baked Bar

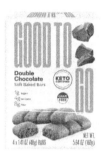

Other Great Products:

Made Good Mixed Berry Granola Bars

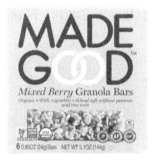

Super Pop Snacks Peanut Butter & Honey Bar

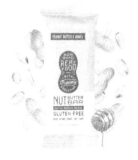

Desserts

Ice Cream Brands

2023 Annual Plant Based Awards

1st Place Winner: So Delicious Ice Cream Coconut Milk Mint Chip

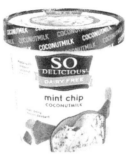

2nd Place Winner: Ben & Jerry's Non Dairy Frozen Dessert Caramel Almond Brittle

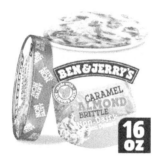

3rd Place Winner: Oatly Chocolate Frozen Dessert

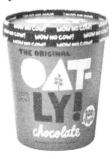

Runner Up:

Coolhaus Tahitian Vanilla Frozen Dessert Sandwich

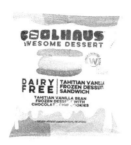

Other Great Products:

NadaMoo! Dairy Free Strawberry Ice Cream

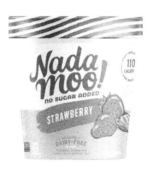

Cosmic Bliss Mint Chip Galactica

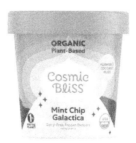

Pie Crust

2022 Annual Plant Based Awards

1st Place Winner: Fifty50 Foods Sugar Free Ready to Eat Graham Cracker Pie Crust

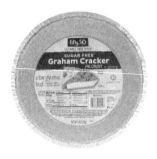

2nd Place Winner: Kbosh Keto Crusts

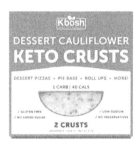

3rd Place Winner: Sooo Ketolicious Premium Keto Pie Crust

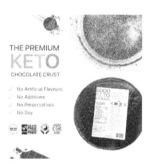

Runner Up:

Diamond Pecan Pie Crust

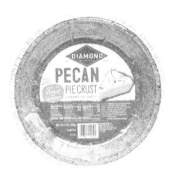

Ready Made Desserts

2023 Annual Plant Based Awards

1st Place Winner: Blissfully Better Organic Dark Chocolate BonBons

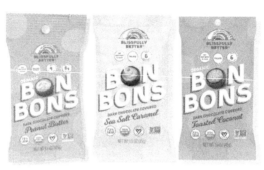

2nd Place Winner: Ben & Jerry's Cherry Garcia Non Dairy Frozen Dessert

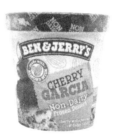

3rd Place Winner: Oatly Strawberry Frozen Dessert

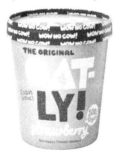

Runner Up:

Better Bites Birthday Do Bites

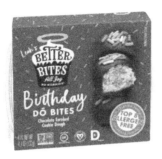

Other Great Products:

Better Bites Mostess Mini-cupcakes

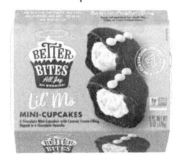

Cosmic Bliss Frozen Dessert Sandwich (Gluten Free)

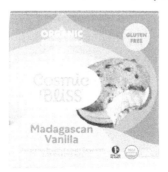

Beverages

Creamers

2023 Annual Plant Based Awards

1st Place Winner: Califia Farms Unsweetened Oat Creamer

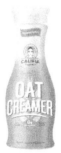

2nd Place Winner: So Delicious Organic Coconutmilk Creamer French Vanilla

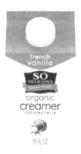

3rd Place Winner: Laird Superfood Unsweetened Superfood Creamer

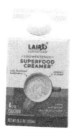

Runner Up:

Anthony's Organic Coconut Creamer

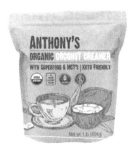

Other Great Creamers:

Nut Pods Almond + Coconut Creamer

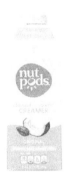

Silk Soy Creamer – Original Flavor

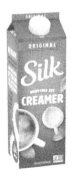

Ready-to-Drink Protein Shakes

2023 Annual Plant Based Awards

1st Place Winner: Orgain Plant-Based Protein Shake - Chocolate

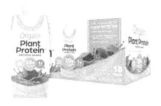

2nd Place Winner: OWYN Vanilla Plant Based Protein Shake

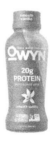

3rd Place Winner: Evolve Classic Chocolate Protein Shake

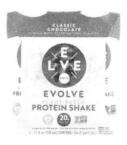

Runner Up:

Forager Project Organic Dairy-Free Nuts & Cocoa Protein Plant Shake

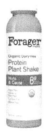

Other Great Protein Shakes:

Koia Protein Cacao Bean

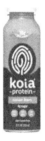

Designs for Health VegeMeal

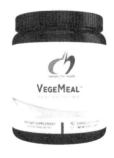

Dry Mixes

Bread Mixes

2023 Annual Plant Based Awards

1st Place Winner: No Sugar Aloud Low Carb Banana Bread Mix

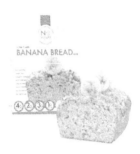

2nd Place Winner: Extra White Gold Gluten Free Bread Flour Blend

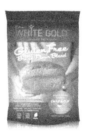

3rd Place Winner: Truly AIP Rustic Bread Mix

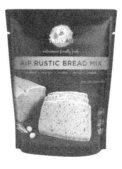

Runner Up:

Simple Mills Almond Flour Baking Mix

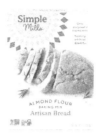

Other Great Products:

Gf Jules Bread mix

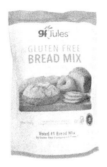

Legit Blonde Sandwich Bread Mix

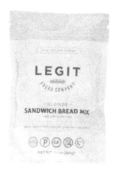

Brownie Mixes

2023 Annual Plant Based Awards

1st Place Winner: Better Batter Fudge Brownie Mix

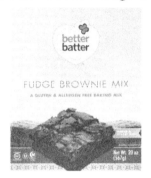

2nd Place Winner: Julie's Real Certified USDA Organic Paleo Dark Chocolate Brownie Mix

Mix

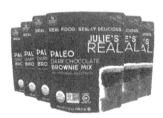

3rd Place Winner: Renewal Mill Dark Chocolate Brownie

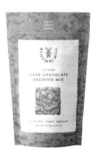

Runner Up:

Lakanto Sugar-free Brownie Mix.

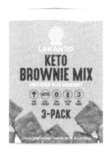

Other Great Products:

Simple Mills Almond Flour Brownie Mix

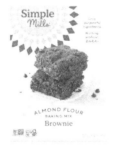

King Arthur Gluten Free Fudge Brownie Mix

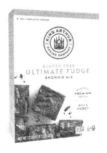

Cake Mixes

2023 Annual Plant Based Awards

1st Place Winner: Better Batter Chocolate Cake Mix

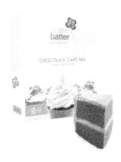

2nd Place Winner: Better Batter Yellow Cake Mix

3rd Place Winner: Miss Jones Baking Chocolate Organic Cake and Cupcake Mix

Runner Up:

Gf Jules Cake Mix

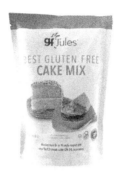

Other Great Products:

Simple Mills Vanilla Almond Flour Baking Mix

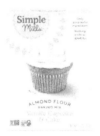

King Arthur Gluten Free Chocolate Cake Mix

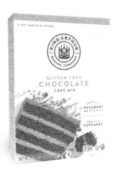

Cookie Mixes

2023 Annual Plant Based Awards

1st Place Winner: gfJules Graham Cracker - Gingerbread Mix

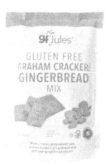

2nd Place Winner: Lakanto Double Chocolate Cookie Mix

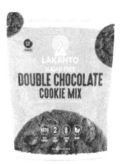

3rd Place Winner: Annie's Organic Cookie Brownie Bar Baking Mix

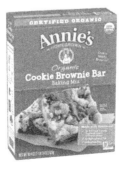

Runner Up:

Foodstirs Keto Chocolate Chip Cookie Mix

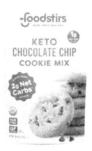

Other Great Products:

Snacktivist Foods - Gluten-Free Chocolate Chip Cookie Baking Mix

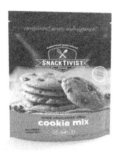

Sweet Loren's Gluten Free Vegan Cookie Dough Mix

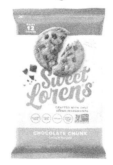

Cornbread Mixes

2023 Annual Plant Based Awards

1st Place Winner: Cup4Cup Gluten Free Cornbread Mix

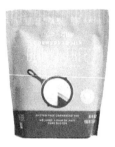

2nd Place Winner: Highkey Bread and Muffin Mix Cornbread

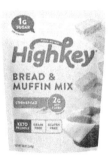

3rd Place Winner: Really Great Food Company – Gluten Free Cornbread Muffin Mix

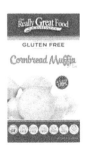

Runner Up:

Good Dee's Corn Bread Baking Mix

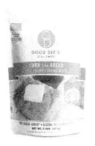

Other Great Products:

gf Jules Cornbread Mix

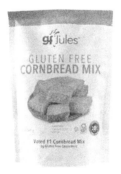

King Arthur Gluten-Free Cornbread and Muffin Mix

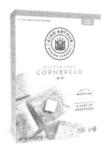

Flours

2023 Annual Plant Based Awards

1st Place Winner: Bob's Red Mill Super-Fine Natural Almond Flour

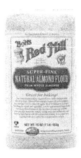

2nd Place Winner: King Arthur Flour Organic All Purpose Flour

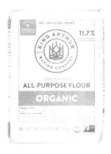

3rd Place Winner: gfJules All Purpose Gluten Free Flour

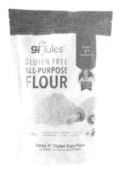

Runner Up:

Better Batter Artisan Flour Blend

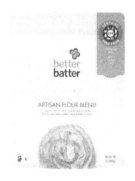

Other Great Products:

Otto's Naturals Cassava Flour

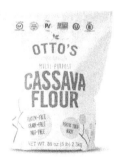

Muffin Mixes

2023 Annual Plant Based Awards

1st Place Winner: Simple Mills Pumpkin Muffin & Bread Almond Flour Mix

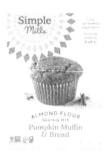

2nd Place Winner: Miss Jones Baking Keto Blueberry Muffin Mix

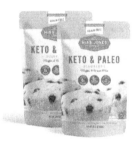

3rd Place Winner: gf Jules Muffin Mix

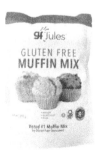

Runner Up:

Lakanto Blueberry Muffin Mix

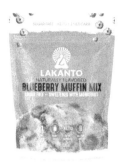

Other Great Products:

Krusteaz Plant Based Blueberry Muffin Mix

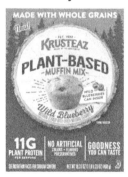

Frozen Foods

Frozen Food

2023 Annual Plant Based Awards

1st Place Winner: Dr. Praeger's Perfect Burgers

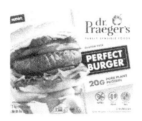

2nd Place Winner: Daiya Foods Pepperoni Style Gluten-free Pizza

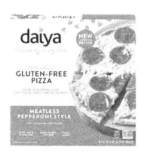

3rd Place Winner: ALDI-exclusive Season's Choice Sweetened Acai Superfruit Packs

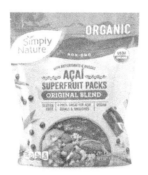

Runner Up:

ALDI-exclusive Season's Choice Unsweetened Acai Super-fruit Packs

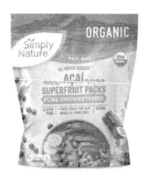

Other Great Products:

Feel Good Foods Vegetable Potstickers

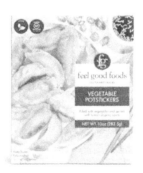

Frozen Meals

2023 Annual Plant Based Awards

1st Place Winner: Amy's Kitchen Pad Thai, GF and Dairy Free

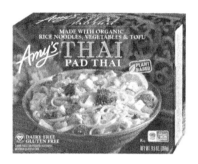

2nd Place Winner: Gardein Italian Style Skillet Meal

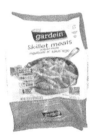

3rd Place Winner: Purple Carrot Sweet Corn Elote Bowl

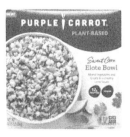

Runner Up:

Gardein Chick'n Florentino Skillet Meal

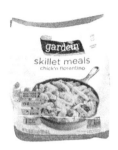

Other Great Products:

Amy's Bean & Rice Burrito, Gluten Free, Non-Dairy

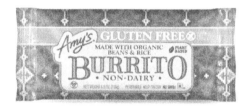

Frozen Pizza

2023 Annual Plant Based Awards

1st Place Winner: Amy's Kitchen Vegan Margherita Pizza

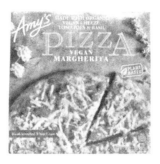

2nd Place Winner: Daiya Foods Pepperoni Style Gluten-free

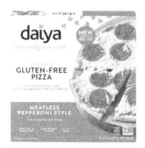

3rd Place Winner: American Flatbread Vegan Harvest Flatbread

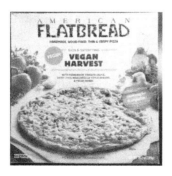

Runner Up:

Sweet Earth Veggie Lover's Frozen Pizza

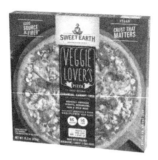

Other Great Products:

Pizza Oggi Siciliana Plant Based Crust Cauliflower

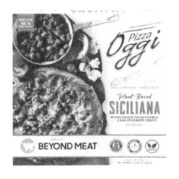

Books

Books

2023 Annual Plant Based Awards

1st Place Winner: The Omnivore's Dilemma: A Natural History of Four Meals by Michael Pollan

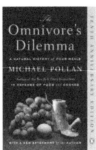

2nd Place Winner: This Is Your Mind on Plants Hardcover by Michael Pollan

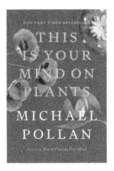

3rd Place Winner: Fiber Fueled: The Plant-Based Gut Health Program for Losing Weight, Restoring Your Health, and Optimizing Your Microbiome by Will Bulsiewicz MD

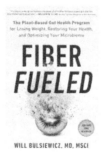

Runner Up:

The Plant-Based Athlete: A Game-Changing Approach to Peak Performance by Matt Frazier

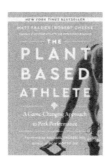

Other Great Books:

Living among Meat Eaters: The Vegetarian's Survival Handbook by Carol Adams

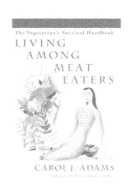

Children's Books

2023 Annual Plant Based Awards

1st Place Winner: The Vegan Cookbook for Kids: Easy Plant-Based Recipes for Young Chefs by Barb Musick

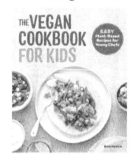

2nd Place Winner: Linus the Vegetarian T. rex by Robert Neubecker

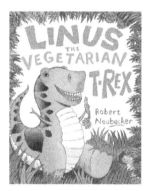

3rd Place Winner: V Is for Vegan: The ABCs of Being Kind by Ruby Roth

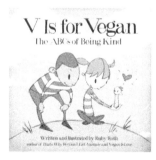

Runner Up:

That's Why We Don't Eat Animals: A Book About Vegans, Vegetarians, and All Living Things by Ruby Roth

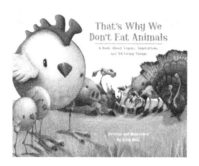

Other Great Books:

The Help Yourself Cookbook for Kids: 60 Easy Plant-Based Recipes Kids Can Make to Stay Healthy and Save the Earth

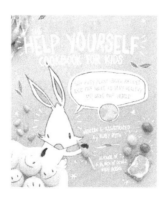

Cookbooks

2023 Annual Plant Based Awards

1st Place Winner: Fast Easy Cheap Vegan: 101 Recipes You Can Make in 30 Minutes or Less, for $10 or Less, and with 10 Ingredients or Less! by Sam Turnbull

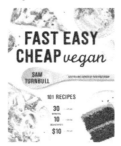

2nd Place Winner: The Complete Plant Based Cookbook For Beginners: 550 Plant-Based Healthy Diet Recipes To Cook Quick & Easy Meals by Jordan Worthen

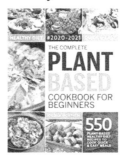

3rd Place Winner: The Vegan Instant Pot Cookbook: Wholesome, Indulgent Plant-Based Recipes by Nisha Vora

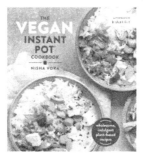

Runner Up:

Plant Over Processed: 75 Simple & Delicious Plant-Based Recipes for Nourishing Your Body and Eating From the Earth by Andrea Hannemann

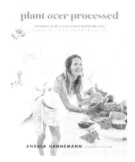

Other Great Cookbooks:

Vegan, but with Soul by Darius Williams

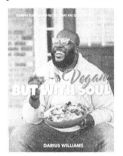

2023 Whole Food Plant-Based Cookbook: 365 Days of Super Easy Plant-Based Recipes for Clean & Healthy Eating | 28 Day Meal Plan Included

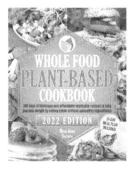

Media

Blogs

2022 Annual Plant Based Awards

1st Place Winner: Plant Based on a Budget plantbasedonabudget.com

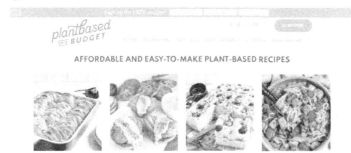

2nd Place Winner: Love & Lemons -   loveandlemons.com

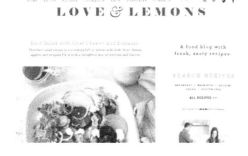

3rd Place Winner: Running on Real Food - runningonrealfood.com

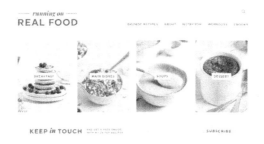

Runner Up:

The First Mess -   thefirstmess.com

HOME   RECIPE SEARCH   COOKBOOK   CATEGORIES   ABOUT   CONTACT

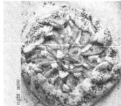
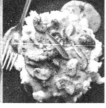

50+ Vegan
Holiday Recipes

All of my best vegan holiday recipes for
entertaining! A bunch of delicious, mostly
gluten-free holiday-appropriate dishes for
your meal planning inspiration - whether
you're gathering with the extended family or

Other Great Blogs:

Jessie May - jessie-may.com

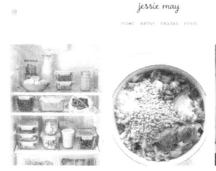
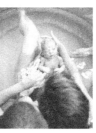

VeganRicha.com

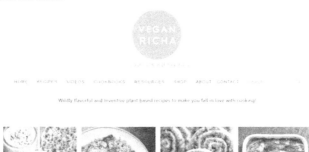

Mobile Apps

2023 Annual Plant Based Awards

1st Place Winner: Oh She Glows

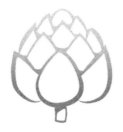

2nd Place Winner: Food Monster

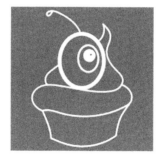

3rd Place Winner: BevVeg

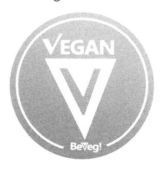

Runner Up:

Vegan Additives

Other Great Apps:

Happy Cow

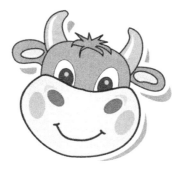

Forks Over Knives

Online Resources

2023 Annual Plant Based Awards

1st Place Winner: Thrive thrivemagazine.com

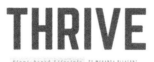

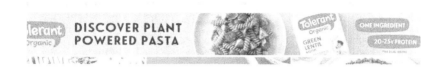

2nd Place Winner: Vegan Outreach veganoutreach.org

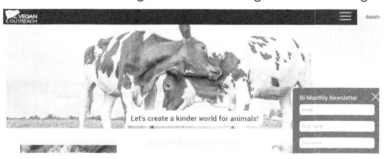

3rd Place Winner: Plant Based Research plant-basedresearch.org

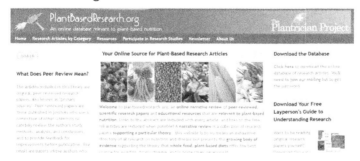

Runner Up:

The Vegetarian Resource Group vrg.org

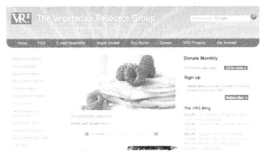

Other Great Resources:

Ocean Robbins foodrevolution.org

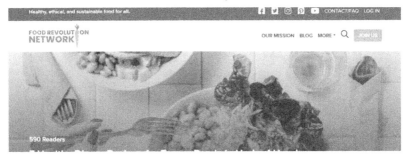

Forks Over Knives

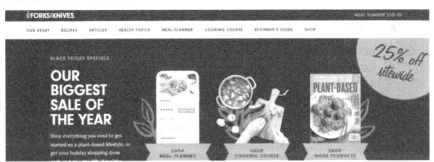

Podcasts

2023 Annual Plant Based Awards

1st Place Winner: Ordinary Vegan Podcast

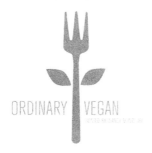

2nd Place Winner: The Plant Proof Podcast with Simon Hill

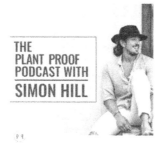

3rd Place Winner: Brown Vegan Podcast

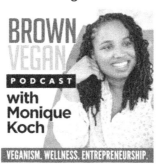

Runner Up:

PLANTSTRONG

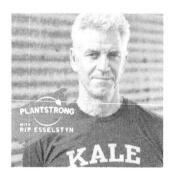

Other Great Podcasts:

No Meat Athlete Radio

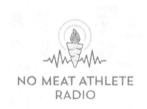

Websites

2022 Annual Plant Based Awards

1st Place Winner: Plant Based Research

plantbasedresearch.org

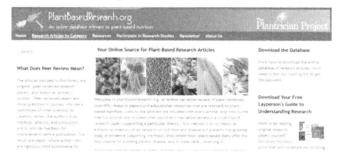

2nd Place Winner: Thrive thrivemagazine.com

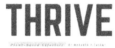

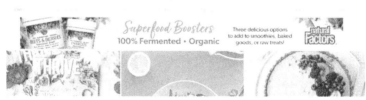

3rd Place Winner: Vegan Outreach veganoutreach.org

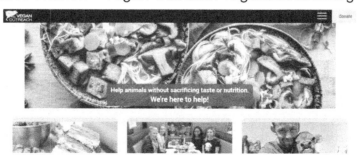

Runner Up:

The Vegetarian Resource Group vrg.org

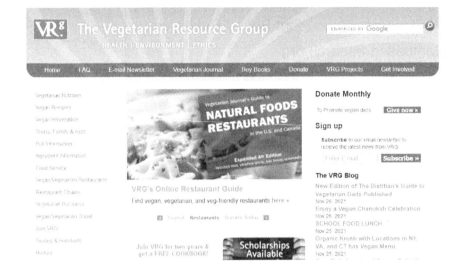

Forks over Knifes forksoverknives.com

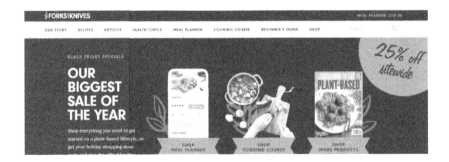

Other

Butter

2023 Annual Plant Based Awards

1st Place Winner: Earth Balance Original Buttery Spread

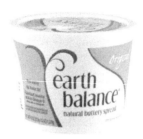

2nd Place Winner: Miyoko's Creamery Unsalted Cultured Vegan Butter

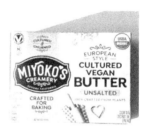

3rd Place Winner: Kite Hill Plant-Based Butter

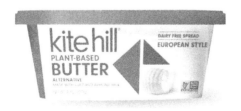

Runner Up:

Milkadamia Salted Buttery Spread

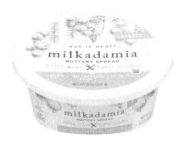

Other Great Products:

Country Crock Plant Butter with Olive Oil

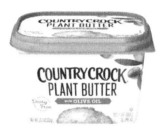

Melt Organic

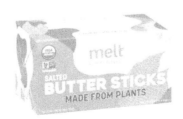

Cheese

2023 Annual Plant Based Awards

1st Place Winner: Violife Cheddar Style Slices

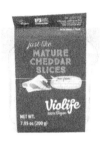

2nd Place Winner: Miyoko's Creamery Vegan Cheese No. 7 Aged English Sharp Farmhouse Cheese Wheel

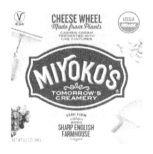

3rd Place Winner: 365 by Whole Foods Market Non-dairy Mozzarella Cheese Shreds

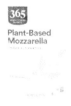

Runner Up:

Follow Your Heart Parmesan - Shredded

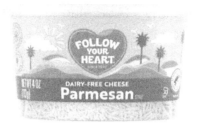

Other Great Products:

Miyoko's Fresh Vegan Mozzarella

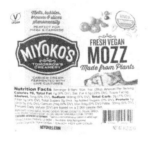

Field Roast Chao Smoked Original Slices

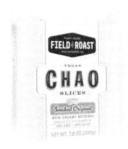

Comfort Foods

2023 Annual Plant Based Awards

1st Place Winner: Amy's Rice Mac & Cheeze, Vegan

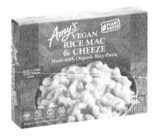

2nd Place Winner: Oatly Strawberry Non-dairy frozen dessert

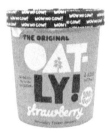

3rd Place Winner: Amy's Organic Gluten Free Medium Chili

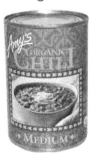

Runner Up:

Kevin's Natural Foods Cauli Mac & Cheese

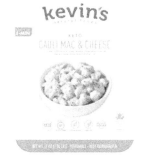

Other Great Products:

Sunscoop Vanilla Tart Cream

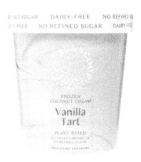

Egg Replacement

2023 Annual Plant Based Awards

1st Place Winner: Bob's Red Mill Egg Substitute

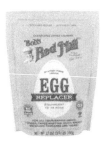

2nd Place Winner: JUST Egg made from plants

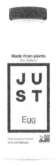

3rd Place Winner: Vegan Egg Replacer by Ener-G

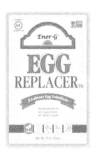

Runner Up:

OGGS

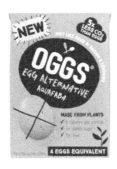

Other Great Products:

Follow Your Heart Vegan Egg

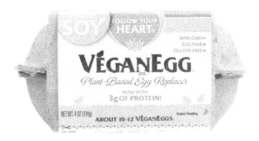

Meat Replacement

2023 Annual Plant Based Awards

1st Place Winner: Beyond Meat Beyond Burger

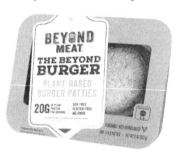

2nd Place Winner: ALDI-exclusive Earth Grown Chicken-less Tenders

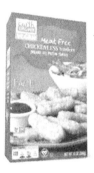

3rd Place Winner: ALDI-exclusive Earth Grown Chickenless Patties

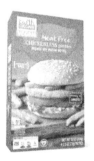

Runner Up:

ALDI-exclusive Earth Grown Classic Meatless Meatballs

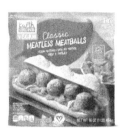

Other Great Products:

ALDI-exclusive Earth Grown Meat Free Turkey Breast

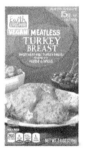

Field Roast Plant-Based Buffalo Wings

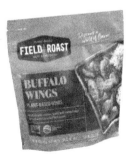

ALDI-exclusive Earth Grown Zesty Meatless Meatballs

Gardein Chipotle Lime Crispy Fingers

New Products

2023 Annual Plant Based Awards

1st Place Winner: San-J Organic Tamari Lite Soy Sauce 50% less sodium

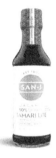

2nd Place Winner: Bakery on Main Bakeshop Bliss Monster Cookie Decadent Granola

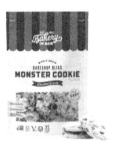

3rd Place Winner: OmniPork

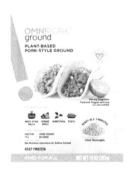

Runner Up:

Dandies Maple Marshmallows

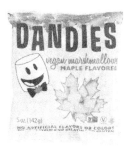

Other Great Products:

Wholly Veggie Mozzarella Style Sticks

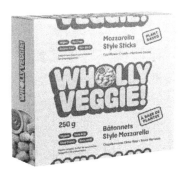

Tofu

2023 Annual Plant Based Awards

1st Place Winner: 365 by Whole Foods Market Organic Silken Tofu

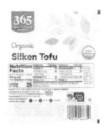

2nd Place Winner: Morinaga Mori-Nu Firm Silken Tofu

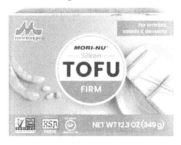

3rd Place Winner: Wildwood Organic Extra Firm Tofu

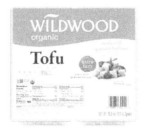

Runner Up:

Hodo Organic Firm Tofu

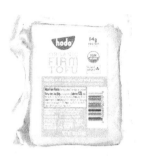

Other Great Products:

House Brand Premium Firm Tofu

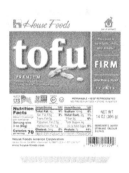

Cosmetics

2023 Annual Plant Based Awards

1st Place Winner: E.L.F. Cosmetics

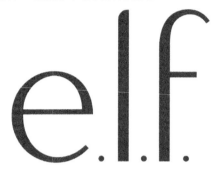

2nd Place Winner: Pacifica

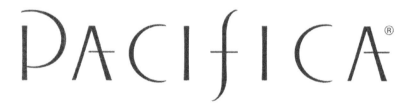

3rd Place Winner: Bite Beauty

Runner Up:

Milk Makeup

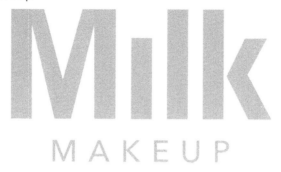

Other Great Products:

KVD Vegan Beauty

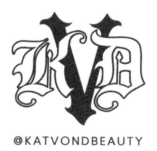

@KATVONDBEAUTY

Hourglass Cosmetics

HOURGLASS

Pasta, Sides, Soup & Sauces

Macaroni and Cheese

2023 Annual Plant Based Awards

1st Place Winner: Annie's Homegrown Mac & Cheese Cheddar Deluxe - Vegan

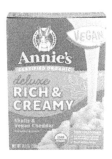

2nd Place Winner: Banza Plant-Based Chickpea Mac & Cheese

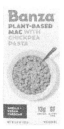

3rd Place Winner: Modern Table Classic Cheddar Mac & Cheese

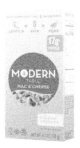

Runner Up:

PASTABILITIES Organic Pasta Ruffles Mac 'N Cheese

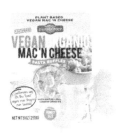

Other Great Products:

Daiya Cheddar Style Mac & Cheeze

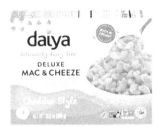

Eat Howl Dairy-Free Creamy Cashew Vegan Mac & Cheese, Classic Sharp Cheddar

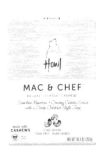

Pastas

2023 Annual Plant Based Awards

1st Place Winner: Banza Chickpea Linguine Pasta

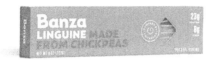

2nd Place Winner: Rao's Homemade Pasta Penne Pasta

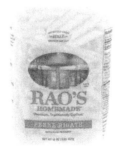

3rd Place Winner: Solely Organic Spaghetti Squash Pasta

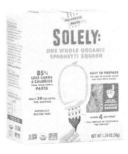

Runner Up:

Sfoglini Trumpets Pasta

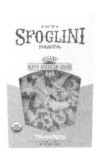

Other Great Products:

Barilla Gluten Free Penne Pasta

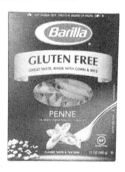

NoNo Pasta Gourmet Superfood with Adaptogens Turmeric-Hemp Fusilli

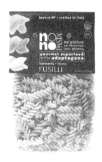

Condiments

2023 Annual Plant Based Awards

1st Place Winner: Primal Kitchen Avocado Oil Mayo 365 by

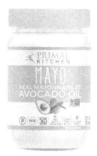

2nd Place Winner: Plant Perfect Vegan Mayo

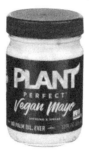

3rd Place Winner: Noble Made by the New Primal Tomato Ketchup

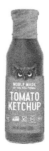

Runner Up:

Follow Your Heart Soy-Free Vegenaise

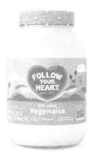

Other Great Products:

Whole Foods Market German Mustard

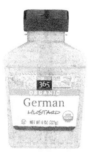

Hidden Valley Plant Powered Ranch

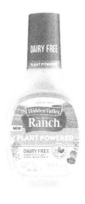

Dips and Spreads

2023 Annual Plant Based Awards

1st Place Winner: Ithaca Hummus Lemon Garlic Hummus

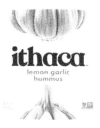

2nd Place Winner: Bitchin' Sauce Chocolate Dip

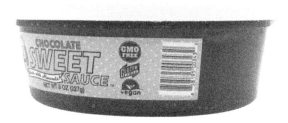

3rd Place Winner: Bitchin' Sauce Chipotle

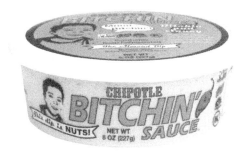

Runner Up:

Plant Perks Garlic & Herb Cheeze Spread

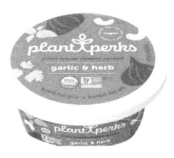

Other Great Products:

Primal Kitchen Ranch Dip Made With Avocado Oil

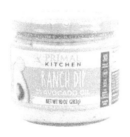

Dressing

2023 Annual Plant Based Awards

1st Place Winner: Newman's Own Olive Oil & Vinegar Dressing

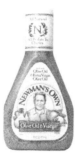

2nd Place Winner: Annie's Homegrown Organic Goddess Dressing

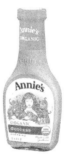

3rd Place Winner: Trader Joe's Green Goddess Salad Dressing,

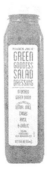

Runner Up:

Fody™ SALAD DRESSING Caesar

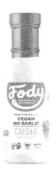

Other Great Products:

Daiya Gluten Free Dairy Free Ranch Dressing

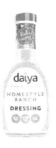

Follow Your Heart Ranch Dressing

Sauces

2023 Annual Plant Based Awards

1st Place Winner: San-J Organic Tamari Gluten Free Soy Sauce

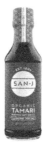

2nd Place Winner: Primal Kitchen Steak Sauce and Marinade

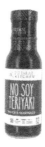

3rd Place Winner: Ocean's Halo Organic Soy-Free Teriyaki Sauce

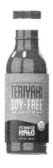

Runner Up:

Noble Made by the New Primal Mild Buffalo Dipping & Wing Sauce

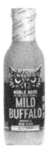

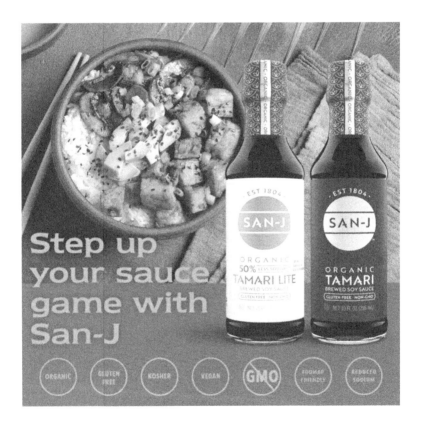

Soup

2023 Annual Plant Based Awards

1st Place Winner: Amy's Kitchen No Chicken Noodle Soup

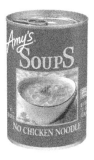

2nd Place Winner: Pacific Foods Pacific Thai Sweet Potato Soup

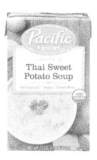

3rd Place Winner: Wolfgang Puck Organic Tortilla Soup

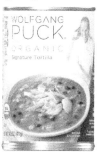

Runner Up:

Dr. McDougall's Right Foods Vegan Pad Thai Noodle Soup

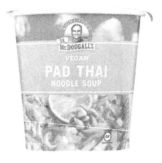

Other Great Products:

Wolfgang Puck Organic Garden Vegetable Soup

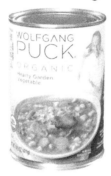

Stuffing

2023 Annual Plant Based Awards

1st Place Winner: Arrowhead Mills Organic Savory Herb Stuffing

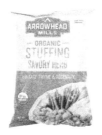

2nd Place Winner: Pepperidge Farm Herb Seasoned Classic Stuffing

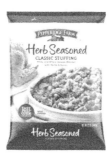

3rd Place Winner: Olivia's Croutons Traditional Stuffing Mix

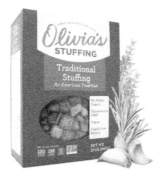

Runner Up:

Aleia's Gluten Free Stuffing

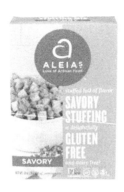

Other Great Products:

Ener G Unseasoned Traditional Stuffing

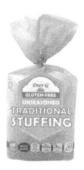

Personalities

Best Plant Based Personality

2023 Annual Plant Based Awards

1st Place Winner: Samira Kazan from AlphaFoodie

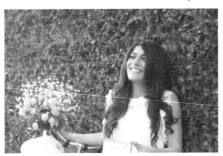

2nd Place Winner: Ella Mills from Deliciously Ella

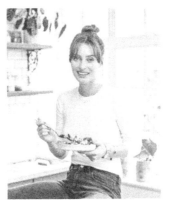

3rd Place Winner: Lauren Toyota from hot for food

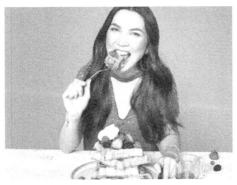

Runner Up: Laird Hamilton from Lairds

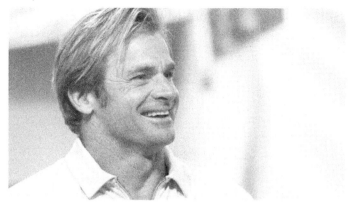

Other great Plant Based people:

Jenn Sebestyen from Veggie Inspired

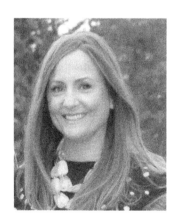

Caitlin Shoemaker from From My Bowl

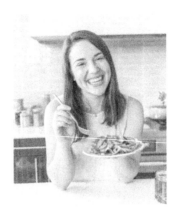

Tabitha Brown

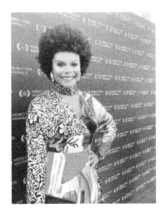

Plant Based Product Registration

By submitting your products into The Plant Based Awards (PBA), you are automatically entering products into the Annual Plant Based Buyers Guide. There are only 10 slots available in each category and we limit brands to 3 submissions per category. If you are a marketer representing multiple brands, this typically will not apply. Slots can fill quickly so we recommend submitting your registration ASAP. The absolute deadline for registration is June 30th however, we cannot guarantee you that the category is already full.

"How do I get into the Plant Based Awards?"

How it works:

1. Fill out the registration form by adding the quantities and product names.

(A free half page ad is given for every 5 products or full-page ad for 10 products.)

2. If wanted, add additional ad space to registration.

3. Email the registration form to Jayme@TheGuidedBuyer.com

4. We will follow up with a confirmation and invoice.

If you have any questions call customer support at 828-455-9734

"Wait, I have tons of questions still"

Most common questions:

Q: I am having a hard time understanding how to submit or products.

A: Using this Registration Form will help. If lost, don't hesitate to call or email. 828-455-9734

Q: What are the image specs you need?

A: Our graphic team just needs images that are PDF, JPEG or PNG at 300 dpi or greater. The team will normally resize images based on the publishing media. Normally the product pictures and descriptions from your website will work just fine.

Full Page Ad Size 384 by 576 px

Half Page Ad Size 384 by 288 px

Q: Is there a word count for product descriptions?

A: No, we normally don't use product descriptions just product names and images.

Q: If we submit 10 products do, we get 1 free full-page ad and 2 free half page ads?

A: Sorry, please choose one or the other. You can always purchase additional ad space.

Q: Can we run a full-page ad without entering the awards program?

A: Yes.

Q: Do we need to send you product samples?

A: No. The community votes for your products.

Q: Will we be in the guide if we don't win an award?

A: Yes, all products submitted will be visible as nominees.

Q: Can we use the LCA Nominee and Winner Badge on our product packaging, website and other related media?

A: Yes, we highly recommend using the badges to differentiate your products from the rest. If you happen to need higher resolution images don't hesitate to ask. Read our media terms here.

Need to talk about your order or have questions? Give us a call.

828-455-9734

or email

Josh@TheGuidedBuyer.com

From our family to yours, have a happy and healthy Plant Based lifestyle.

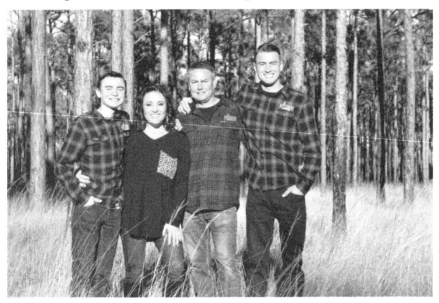

The Schieffer Family

Josh (Dad with Celiac) Chief Marketing Officer

Jayme (Mom) VP Operations

Blake (22)

Jacob (18 Celiac)

Keep up to date with us, the awards, and future buyer guides at TheGuidedBuyer.com

Notes:

Notes:

Notes:

Notes:

COMING SOON - REGISTER NOW

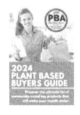

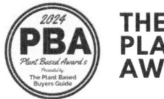

THE 2024
PLANT BASED
AWARDS HOSTED BY
THE GUIDED BUYER.COM

Made in the USA
Las Vegas, NV
26 August 2023

76654822R00095